THE KEYS TO PERFECT HEALTH

ULTIMATE SECRETS ON HOW TO STAY HEALTHY AS A WOMAN

A.G. GIDEON

Table of contents

Chapter 1
Chapter 2
Chapter 3
Chapter 4
Chapter 5

Chapter 1

Birth control

Birth control (contraception) is any method, medicine, or device used to prevent pregnancy. Women can choose from many different types of birth control. Some work better than others at preventing pregnancy. The type of birth control you use depends on your health, your desire to have children now or in the future, and your need to prevent sexually transmitted infections. Your doctor can help you decide which type is best for you right now.

What is the best method of birth control?
There is no "best" method of birth control for every woman. The birth control method that is right for you and your partner depends on many things and may change over time.

Before choosing a birth control method, talk to your doctor or nurse about:

Whether you want to get pregnant soon, in a few years, or never
How well each method works to prevent pregnancy
Possible side effects
How often do you have sex
The number of sex partners you have
Your overall health
How comfortable you are with using the method (For example, can you remember to take a pill every day? Will you have to ask your partner to put on a condom each time?)
Learn about types of birth control that you or your partner can use to prevent pregnancy.

Keep in mind that even the most effective birth control methods can fail. But your chances of getting pregnant are lower if you use a more effective method.

What are the different types of birth control?
Women can choose from many different types of birth control methods. These include, in order of most effective to least effective at preventing pregnancy:

Female and male sterilization (female tubal ligation or occlusion, male vasectomy) — Birth control that prevents pregnancy for the rest of your life through surgery or a medical procedure. Long-acting reversible contraceptives or "LARC" methods (intrauterine devices, hormonal implants) — Birth control your doctor inserts one time and you do not have to remember to use birth control every day or month. LARCs last for 3 to 10 years, depending on the method.

Short-acting hormonal methods (pill, mini pills, patch, shot, vaginal ring) — Birth control your doctor prescribes that you remember to take every day or month. The shot requires you to get a shot from your doctor every 3 months.

Barrier methods (condoms, diaphragms, sponge, cervical cap) — Birth control you use each time you have sex.

Natural rhythm methods — Not using a type of birth control but instead avoiding sex and/or using birth control only on the days when you are most fertile (most likely to get pregnant). An ovulation home test kit or a fertility monitor can help you find your most fertile days.

How can I compare the different types of birth control?

Types of birth control

Method

Number of pregnancies per 100 women within their first year of typical use1

Side effects and risks*

*These are not all of the possible side effects and risks. Talk to your doctor or nurse for more information.

How often do you have to take or use

Abstinence (no sexual contact)

Unknown

(0 for perfect use)

No medical side effects

No action is required, but it does take willpower. You may want to have a backup birth control method, such as condoms.

Permanent sterilization surgery for women (tubal ligation, "getting your tubes tied")

Less than 1

Possible pain during recovery (up to 2 weeks)
Bleeding or other complications from surgery
Less common risk includes ectopic (tubal) pregnancy
No action is required after surgery

Permanent sterilization implant for women (Essure®)

The Essure® birth control device will no longer be sold or distributed in the United States after December 31, 2018.

Less than 1

Pain during the insertion of Essure; some pain during recovery
Cramping, vaginal bleeding, and back pain during recovery
The implant may move out of place
Less common but serious risk includes ectopic (tubal) pregnancy
No action is required after surgery

Permanent sterilization surgery for men (vasectomy)

Less than 1

Pain during recovery
Complications from surgery
No action is required after surgery

Implantable rod (Implanon®, Nexplanon®)

Less than 1

Headache
Irregular periods
Weight gain
Sore breasts
Less common risk includes difficulty in removing the implant
No action is required for up to 3 years before removing or replacing

Copper intrauterine device (IUD) (ParaGard®)

Less than 1

Cramps for a few days after insertion
Missed periods, bleeding between periods, heavier periods
Less common but serious risks include pelvic inflammatory disease and the IUD being expelled from the uterus or going through the wall of the uterus.
No action is required for up to 10 years before removing or replacing

Hormonal intrauterine devices (IUDs) (Liletta, Mirena®, and Skyla®)

Less than 1

Irregular periods, lighter or missed periods
Ovarian cysts
Less common but serious risks include pelvic inflammatory disease and the IUD being expelled from the uterus or going through the wall of the uterus.
No action is required for 3 to 5 years, depending on the brand, before removing or replacing

Shot/injection (Depo-Provera®)

6

Bleeding between periods, missed periods
Weight gain
Changes in mood
Sore breasts
Headaches
Bone loss with long-term use (bone loss may be reversible once you stop using this type of birth control)
Get a new shot every 3 months

Oral contraceptives, combination hormones ("the pill")

9

Headache
Upset stomach
Sore breasts
Changes in your period
Changes in mood
Weight gain
High blood pressure
Less common but serious risks include blood clots, stroke, and heart attack; the risk is higher in smokers and women older than 35
Take it at the same time every day

Oral contraceptives, progestin-only pill ("mini-pill")

9

Spotting or bleeding between periods
Weight gain
Sore breasts
Headache
Nausea
Take it at the same time every day

Skin patch
(Xulane®)

9

May be less effective in women weighing 198 pounds or more2

Skin irritation
Upset stomach
Changes in your period
Changes in mood
Sore breasts
Headache
Weight gain
High blood pressure
Less common but serious risks include blood clots, stroke, and heart attack; the risk is higher in smokers and women older than 35
Wear for 21 days, remove for 7 days, and replace with a new patch

Vaginal ring (NuvaRing®)

9

Headache
Upset stomach
Sore breasts
Vaginal irritation and discharge
Changes in your period
High blood pressure
Less common but serious risks include blood clots, stroke, and heart attack; the risk is higher in smokers and women older than 35
Wear for 21 days, remove for 7 days, and replace with a new ring

Diaphragm with spermicide (Koromex®, Ortho-Diaphragm®)

12

If you gain or lose more than 15 pounds, or have a baby, have your doctor check you to make sure the diaphragm still fits.

Irritation
Allergic reactions
Urinary tract infection (UTI)

Vaginal infections
Rarely, toxic shock if left in for more than 24 hours
Using a spermicide often might increase your risk of getting HIV
Insert each time you have sex

Sponge with spermicide (Today Sponge®)

12

(among women who have never given birth before)

or

24

(among women who have given birth)3

Irritation
Allergic reactions
Rarely, toxic shock if left in for more than 24 hours
Using a spermicide often might increase your risk of getting HIV
Insert each time you have sex

Cervical cap with spermicide (FemCap®)

233

Vaginal irritation or odor
Urinary tract infections (UTIs)
Allergic reactions
Rarely, toxic shock if left in for more than 48 hours
Using a spermicide often might increase your risk of getting HIV
Insert each time you have sex

Male condom

18

Irritation
The condom may tear, break or slip off
Allergic reactions to latex condoms
Use each time you have sex

Female condom

21

Irritation
The condom may tear or slip out
Allergic reaction
Use each time you have sex

Withdrawal — when a man takes his penis out of a woman's vagina (or "pulls out") before he ejaculates (has an orgasm or "comes")

22

Sperm can be released before the man pulls out, putting you at risk for pregnancy
Use each time you have sex

Natural family planning (rhythm method)

24

Can be hard to know the days you are most fertile (when you need to avoid having sex or use backup birth control)
Depending on the method used, takes planning each month

Spermicide alone

28

Works best if used along with a barrier method, such as a diaphragm

Irritation
Allergic reactions
Urinary tract infection
Frequent use of a spermicide might increase your risk of getting HIV
Use each time you have sex

Which types of birth control help prevent sexually transmitted infections (STIs)?
Only two types can protect you from STIs, including HIV: male condoms and female condoms.4

While condoms are the best way to prevent STIs if you have sex, they are not the most effective type of birth control. If you have sex, the best way to prevent both STIs and pregnancy is to use what is called "dual protection." Dual protection means you use a condom to prevent STIs each time you have sex, and at the same time, you use a more effective form of birth control, such as an IUD, implant, or shot.

Which types of birth control can I get without a prescription?
You can buy these types of birth control over the counter at a drugstore or supermarket:

Male condoms
Female condoms
Sponges
Spermicides
Emergency contraception (EC) pills. Plan B One-Step® and its generic versions are available in drugstores and some supermarkets to anyone, without a prescription. However, you should not use EC as your regular birth control because it does not work as well as regular birth control. EC is meant to be used only when your regular birth control does not work for some unexpected reason.
Which types of birth control do I have to see my doctor to get?
You need a prescription for these types of birth control:

Oral contraceptives: the pill and the mini-pill (in some states, birth control pills are now available without a prescription, through the pharmacy)
Patch
Vaginal ring
Diaphragms (your doctor or nurse needs to fit one to the shape of your vagina)
Shot/injection (you get the shot at your doctor's office or family planning clinic)
Cervical cap
Implantable rod (inserted by a doctor in the office or clinic)
IUD (inserted by a doctor in the office or clinic)
You will need surgery or a medical procedure for:

Female sterilization (tubal ligation)
Male sterilization (vasectomy)
Tubal implant (Essure®)
Please note that Essure® will not be sold or distributed in the United States after December 31, 2018.

How does birth control work?
Birth control works to prevent pregnancy in different ways, depending upon the type of birth control you choose:

Female or male sterilization surgery prevents the sperm from reaching the egg by cutting or damaging the tubes that carry sperm (in men) or eggs (in women).
Long-acting reversible contraceptives or "LARC" methods (intrauterine devices, hormonal implants) prevent your ovaries from releasing eggs, prevent sperm from getting to the egg, or make implantation of the egg in the uterus (womb) unlikely.
Short-acting hormonal methods, such as the pill, mini-pill, patch, shot, and vaginal ring, prevent your ovaries from releasing eggs or prevent sperm from getting to the egg.

Barrier methods, such as condoms, diaphragms, sponges, and cervical caps, prevent sperm from getting to the egg.

Natural rhythm methods involve avoiding sex or using other forms of birth control on the days when you are most fertile (most likely to get pregnant).

Are birth control pills safe?

Yes, hormonal birth control methods, such as the pill, are safe for most women. Today's birth control pills have lower doses of hormones than in the past. This has lowered the risk of side effects and serious health problems.

Today's birth control pills can have health benefits for some women, such as a lower risk of some kinds of cancer.5 Also, different brands and types of birth control pills (and other forms of hormonal birth control) can increase your risk for some health problems and side effects. Side effects can include weight gain, headaches, irregular bleeding, breast tenderness, and mood changes.

Talk to your doctor about whether hormonal birth control is right for you.

Does birth control raise my risk for health problems?

It can, depending on your health and the type of birth control you use. Talk to your doctor to find the birth control method that is right for you.

Different forms of birth control have different health risks and side effects. Some birth control methods that increase your risk for health problems include:

Hormonal birth control. Combination birth control pills (birth control with both estrogen and progesterone) and some other forms of hormonal birth control, such as the vaginal ring or skin patch, may raise your risk for blood clots and high blood pressure. Blood clots and high blood pressure can cause a heart attack or stroke. A blood clot in the legs can also go to your lungs, causing serious damage or even death. These are serious side effects of hormonal birth control, but they are rare.

Spermicides (used alone or with the cervical cap, diaphragm, or sponge). Spermicides that have nonoxynol-9 can irritate the vagina. This can raise your risk of getting HIV. Use spermicides with nonoxynol-9 only if you are in a monogamous relationship (you have sex only with each other) with a man you know is HIV-negative. Also, medicines for vaginal yeast infections may make spermicides less effective.

Intrauterine devices (IUDs). IUDs can slightly raise your risk of an ectopic pregnancy. Ectopic pregnancies happen when a fertilized egg implants somewhere outside of the uterus (womb), usually in one of the fallopian tubes. An ectopic pregnancy is a serious medical problem that should be treated as soon as possible. IUDs also have a very rare but serious risk of infection or puncture of the uterus.

What are the health risks for smokers who use birth control?

If you smoke and are 35 or older, you should not use hormonal birth control. Smoking tobacco and using hormonal birth control raises your risk for blood clots and high blood pressure.

Smoking and high blood pressure are risk factors for a heart attack or stroke. The risk of a heart attack or stroke also goes up as you age.

Can birth control help with my painful or heavy periods?
Maybe. Research shows that hormonal birth control, such as the pill, patch, shot, ring, implantable rod, and hormonal IUD, may help with heavy, painful, or long-term bleeding. These methods can also help you have lighter, shorter periods.6

What are some other benefits of hormonal birth control?
Research shows that other benefits of hormonal birth control may include:6,7

More regular and lighter periods
Fewer menstrual cramps
Less acne
Lower risk of the ovary, endometrial (uterus), and colon cancers, pelvic inflammatory disease (PID), non cancerous ovarian cysts, and iron-deficiency anemia
Read more about how birth control can help with the following health problems:

Ovarian cysts
Endometriosis
Polycystic ovary syndrome
Uterine fibroids
What do I do if I miss a day taking the pill?
Follow the instructions that came with your birth control about using backup birth control (such as a condom and spermicide). You also can follow these recommendations from the Centers for Disease Control and Prevention.1

If you are late or miss a day taking your pill:

Take the late or missed pill as soon as possible.
Continue taking the rest of your pills at your normal time, even if it means taking two pills on the same day.
You do not need other forms of birth control, such as a condom unless you need to protect against STIs.
If you miss two or more days in a row:

Take only the most recent missed pill as soon as possible.
Continue taking the rest of your pills at your normal time, even if it means taking two pills on the same day.
Use backup birth control, such as a condom and spermicide, or do not have sex until you have taken a pill for seven days in a row.
If you missed pills during days in the last week of active pills (days 15–21 for 28-day pill packs), start a new pack the next day. If you are not able to start a new pack right away, use backup

birth control or avoid sex until hormone pills from a new pack have been taken for 7 days in a row.

Consider emergency contraception if you missed pills during the first week and had sex.

Talk to your doctor if you continue to miss taking your birth control pill or find it hard to take the pill at the same time each day. You may want to consider a different type of birth control, such as an IUD, an implant, a shot, a ring, or a patch that you don't have to remember to take every day.

How effective is the withdrawal method?

Not very! About 22 out of 100 women who use withdrawal as their only form of birth control for a year will get pregnant. See the chart above for how this number compares to other methods of birth control.

Withdrawal is when a man takes his penis out of a woman's vagina ("pulls out") before he ejaculates or "comes" (has an orgasm). This lowers the chance of sperm going to the egg. "Pulling out" can be hard for a man to do. It takes a lot of self-control.

Even if you use withdrawal, sperm can be released before the man pulls out. When a man's penis first becomes erect, some fluid may be on the tip of the penis. This fluid has sperm in it, so you could still get pregnant. Withdrawal also does not protect you from STIs, including HIV.

Does breastfeeding prevent pregnancy?

Breastfeeding can be a short-term method of birth control in very specific situations. The risk of pregnancy is less than 2 in 100 if all three of these describe you:1

You have a baby who is less than 6 months old
and

You exclusively breastfeed, meaning that you only feed your baby your breastmilk all of the time (no formula, no breast milk from other people, and no solid food)
and

You have not gotten a period after childbirth

Talk to your doctor about birth control if you do not want to get pregnant while nursing.

Chapter 2

Breast augmentation

For some women, breast augmentation is a way to feel more confident. For others, it's part of rebuilding the breast for various conditions.

Enhance your appearance if you think your breasts are small or that one is smaller than the other and this impacts how you dress or the type of bra needed to help with the asymmetry
Adjust for a reduction in the size of your breasts after pregnancy or significant weight loss
Correct uneven breasts after breast surgery for other conditions
Improve your self-confidence
Discuss your goals with your plastic surgeon so that you can be realistic about what breast augmentation can do for you.

Request an appointment
Risks
Breast augmentation poses various risks, including:

Scar tissue that distorts the shape of the breast implant (capsular contracture)
Breast pain
Infection
Changes in nipple and breast sensation
Implant position changes
Implant leakage or rupture
Correcting these complications might require more surgery, to either remove or replace the implants.

Breast implant-associated anaplastic large cell lymphoma
The U.S. Food and Drug Administration (FDA) has identified a possible association between breast implants and the development of anaplastic large cell lymphoma (ALCL), an uncommon cancer of the immune system. The condition is known as breast implant-associated anaplastic large cell lymphoma (BIA-ALCL). The FDA believes that women with breast implants that have textured surfaces have a very low but increased risk of developing BIA-ALCL. However, that doesn't mean that these implants cause BIA-ALCL. Further research is needed to understand the relationship between the condition and breast implants.

Breast implant illness
Systemic symptoms — sometimes called breast implant illness — may be associated with breast implants. The exact relationship of these symptoms to breast implants is not clearly understood. Reported signs and symptoms include fatigue, memory loss, skin rash, trouble concentrating and thinking clearly, and joint pain. Removal of the breast implants may reverse

the symptoms. Research to determine the link and the cause is ongoing. Talk to your plastic surgeon if you have breast implants and experience any of these signs and symptoms.

If you notice any changes to your breasts or implants, talk to your doctor. Ongoing follow-up visits and appropriate screening tests can detect and address possible complications related to breast augmentation surgery.

How you prepare
You'll consult with a plastic surgeon about your preferences for the size, feel, and appearance of your breasts. The surgeon will describe specific types of implants — smooth or textured, round or shaped like a teardrop, saline or silicone — as well as options for surgical techniques.

Carefully review written information, such as the patient information from the manufacturer of the implant you'll be getting, and keep copies for your records.

Before you decide to have surgery, consider the following:

Breast implants won't prevent your breasts from sagging. Your plastic surgeon may recommend a breast lift in addition to breast augmentation to correct sagging breasts.
Breast implants aren't guaranteed to last a lifetime. The average life span of an implant is about 10 years. Implant rupture is a possibility. Also, your breasts will continue to age, and factors such as weight gain or weight loss might change the way your breasts look. These issues will likely lead to more surgery.
Mammograms might be more complicated. If you have breast implants, in addition to routine mammograms, you'll need additional, specialized views.
Breast implants might hamper breastfeeding. Some women can successfully breastfeed after breast augmentation. For others, however, breastfeeding is a challenge.
Insurance doesn't cover breast implants. Unless it's medically necessary — such as after a mastectomy for breast cancer — breast augmentation isn't covered by insurance. Be prepared to handle the expenses, including related surgeries or future imaging tests.
You might need additional surgery after breast implant removal. If you decide to have your implants removed, you might need a breast lift or other corrective surgery to help restore your breasts' appearance.
Screening for silicone implant rupture is recommended. The FDA recommends routine monitoring with a breast MRI five to six years after placement to screen for silicone breast implant rupture. Then, a breast MRI is recommended every two to three years. An ultrasound may be an alternative screening method — unless you have symptoms. Talk to your plastic surgeon about the specific type of imaging needed for routine monitoring of your implants.
You might need a baseline mammogram before your surgery. Your doctor might adjust certain medications before the surgery as well. For example, it's important to avoid aspirin or other medications that can increase bleeding.

If you smoke, your surgeon will ask you to stop smoking for a time — about four to six weeks — before and after the surgery.

Arrange for someone to drive you home after the surgery and to stay with you for at least the first night.

What you can expect
Breast augmentation incision sites
Breast augmentation incision sites Enlarge image placement of breast implants
Placement of breast implants Enlarge image
Breast augmentation can be done in a surgical center or hospital outpatient facility. You'll probably go home the same day. The procedure rarely requires a hospital stay.

Sometimes, breast augmentation is done during local anesthesia — you're awake and your breast area is numbed. Often, though, breast augmentation is done during general anesthesia, in which you're asleep for the surgery. Your plastic surgeon will review different anesthesia options with you.

During the procedure
To insert the breast implant, your plastic surgeon will make a single cut (incision) in one of three places:

The crease under your breast (inframammary)
Under your arm (axillary)
Around your nipple (periareolar)
After making an incision, the surgeon will separate your breast tissue from the muscles and connective tissue of your chest. This creates a pocket either behind or in front of the outermost muscle of the chest wall (pectoral muscle). The surgeon will insert the implant into this pocket and center it behind your nipple.

Saline implants are inserted empty and then filled with sterile salt water once they're in place. Silicone implants are pre-filled with silicone gel.

When the implant is in place, the surgeon will close the incision — typically with stitches (sutures) — and bandage it with skin adhesive and surgical tape.

After the procedure
Soreness and swelling are likely for a few weeks after surgery. Bruising is possible, too. Expect scars to fade over time but not disappear completely.

While you're healing, it might help to wear a compression bandage or sports bra for extra support and positioning of the breast implants. Your surgeon might prescribe pain medication as well.

Follow your surgeon's instructions about returning to regular activities. If you don't have a physically demanding job, you might be able to return to work within a few weeks. Avoid strenuous activities — anything that could raise your pulse or blood pressure — for at least two weeks. While you're healing, remember that your breasts will be sensitive to physical contact or jarring movements.

If your surgeon used sutures that don't absorb on their own or placed drainage tubes near your breasts, you'll need a follow-up appointment for removal.

If you notice warmth and redness in your breast or you have a fever, you might have an infection. Contact your surgeon as soon as possible. Also, contact your surgeon if you have shortness of breath or chest pain.

Results
Breast augmentation can change the size and shape of your breasts. The surgery might improve your body image and self-esteem. But keep your expectations realistic, and don't expect perfection.

Also, your breasts will continue to age after augmentation. Weight gain or weight loss might change the way your breasts look, too. If you become dissatisfied with the appearance of your breasts, you might need more surgery to correct these issues.

Cholesterol medicine

Which Statin Is Safest?

Statins are a class of medication used to reduce the levels of unhealthy LDL cholesterol in your bloodstream. LDL cholesterol is a waxy, fatty substance that sticks to the blood vessels of your heart and the walls of your arteries. This can make your arteries harden.

It also may form plaques that block the normal flow of blood. If plaques break away from the wall of the artery or blood clots form on them, you can have a heart attack or stroke.

Statins reduce your body's ability to manufacture LDL cholesterol. And they work. Statin therapy reduces the risk of a heart attack or other cardiovascular event by as much as 48 percent trusted Source, depending on the level of risk factors you have. Statins are so effective that nearly 32 million Americans take them.

Which statin should I take?
Statins have been studied exhaustively due to their wide use. Statins are safe for most people, but there are differences between individual statins.

So, which statin is safest? It depends on a variety of factors. Some statins are safer for you if you have certain medical conditions. That is because there are known drug interactions between medications and individual statins.

The amount, or dose, you need for a statin to be effective is a factor, too. Your risk is less with lower doses of most statins.

Fewer side effects
According to a research reviewTrusted Source people who take simvastatin (Zocor) or pravastatin (Pravachol) may experience fewer side effects.

If you have many risk factors
Guidelines issued by the American College of Cardiology and American Heart AssociationTrusted Source indicate that the benefits of a high-intensity statin outweigh the risks if:

you have heart disease associated with hardening of the arteries (atherosclerosis) and are 75 years of age or lower

your LDL cholesterol level is 190 mg/dL or greater

you have diabetes and high cholesterol levels and other risk factors for cardiovascular disease

If you need high-intensity statin therapy, your doctor is likely to prescribe atorvastatin (Lipitor) or rosuvastatin (Crestor).

If you take azole antifungal medication
Azole antifungal meds are often prescribed for fungal infections such as thrush and vaginal yeast infections. The American Academy of Family Physicians (AAFP) recommends avoiding lovastatin and simvastatin when taking the antifungal drugs itraconazole (Sporanox) and ketoconazole (Xolegel, Extina, Nizoral).

If you take protease inhibitors
If you take protease inhibitors like atazanavir (Reyataz), ritonavir (Norvir), or lopinavir/ritonavir (Kaletra) to treat HIV/AIDS, the AAFP advises that you avoid:

lovastatin (Mevacor, Altoprev)

pitavastatin (Livalo)

simvastatin (Zocor)

If you take macrolide antibiotics
The AAFP recommends avoiding lovastatin (Mevacor, Altoprev) and simvastatin (Zocor) if you are taking macrolide antibiotics for bacterial infections. If you take atorvastatin or pitavastatin, you may need a dose adjustment.

If you take cyclosporine
Cyclosporine (Neoral) is used to treat several conditions, including psoriasis and rheumatoid arthritis. It's also used to prevent organ rejection after transplants. The AAFP recommends avoiding pitavastatin and pravastatin if you are taking cyclosporine. Other statins including atorvastatin, lovastatin, rosuvastatin, and fluvastatin may require dose adjustments.

What's the safety issue?
Only about 3 to 4 percent of people who take statins don't do well on them, Harvard Health Publications report. For some of these individuals, statins aren't effective in lowering cholesterol. Other people experience side effects.

Minor side effects
Common minor side effects include:

diarrhea
constipation
rash
headache
Liver inflammation
In a small number of people, statins cause an increase in enzymes that the liver uses to help digestion. The liver can become inflamed and there's the risk of damage.

Muscle inflammation and pain
Statins can make muscles sore and tender to the touch. Very rarely, a condition called rhabdomyolysis occurs, in which there is serious damage to the muscles. Rhabdomyolysis is most often seen when people have other risk factors for the disorder, which could include reduced thyroid function, liver disease, and slower kidney function.

Fatigue
Statins can also cause fatigue, especially in women. Fatigue seems to be related to exercise, unfortunately. In one studyTrusted Source, researchers found that four in 10 women experienced a decrease in energy and increased fatigue from exercise when they took 20 mg of simvastatin daily. Your doctor should always check out any unexplained fatigue when you take a statin.

Cognitive problems
Some people may experience problems with their memory and concentration. These symptoms are not serious and can be reversed when discontinuing statins or switching to a different statin.

Diabetes risk
Statins may cause an increase in blood sugar levels for some people. This could increase your risk for diabetes.

Kidney risk
If you have kidney disease, you should know that you might need a different dose of statins. Some high-intensity statin doses are too high for those with kidney disease.

You are pregnant or breast-feeding
Statins are not recommended if you are pregnant or breastfeeding.

You might also need to take cholesterol medications to help: Decrease your low-density lipoprotein (LDL) cholesterol, the "bad" cholesterol that increases the risk of heart disease.
What are statins?
Statins are prescription medications that can lower your cholesterol levels. Popular statins include atorvastatin (Lipitor), rosuvastatin (Crestor), and simvastatin (Zocor).

Statins work in two ways. First, they stop the production of cholesterol in your body. Second, they help your body reabsorb the cholesterol that has built plaques in your artery walls. This reduces your risk of blood vessel blockages and heart attacks.

Statins are typically very successful at lowering cholesterol, but they only work as long as you're taking them. Therefore, most people who begin taking statin medication will likely take it for the rest of their lives.

If you've been taking statins and would like to stop, you'll need to do so with your doctor's guidance. This is because it can be dangerous to stop taking statins. These drugs are highly effective in preventing heart problems such as heart attack and stroke. In fact, according to the American Heart Association (AHA)Trusted Source, they can reduce your risk of these and other cholesterol-related problems by as much as 50 percent. The AHA looks at stopping the use of such effective medications as essentially doubling your risk of these health problems.

Read on to learn about how to stop the use of statins safely.

How to safely come off statins
Some people can stop taking statins safely, but it can be especially risky for others. For instance, if you have a history of heart attack or stroke, it's not recommended that you stop taking these drugs. This is because you're more likely to have another such problem when you discontinue statins.

However, if you don't have a history of heart attack or stroke and you want to stop taking statins, your first step should be to talk to your doctor. They can help you find out what your risk factors are, and if stopping statins is a safe move for you.

If your doctor thinks that you could safely stop taking your statin, they can suggest a plan for it. This plan may involve stopping statins entirely, or it may involve reducing your statin usage.

Another option is to continue taking the statin but add a supplement. One of these options is likely to address whatever problems taking statins causes for you.

Stopping statins
If your doctor will be helping you stop taking statins entirely, some options they might suggest include switching to a different drug or adopting certain lifestyle changes.

Switching medications
Your doctor might suggest changing from a statin to a different type of cholesterol medication.

For instance, the American Heart Association (AHA)Trusted Source recommends the following options for people with high cholesterol who cannot take statins:

ezetimibe, another cholesterol medication
a fabric acid supplement such as fenoic acid, which can lower LDL levels and increase HDL levels
a slow-release niacin supplement, which can lower LDL levels, increase HDL levels, and lower triglyceride levels
A different drug may be able to take the place of a statin in keeping your cholesterol levels in a safe range.

Adopting a diet and exercise program
Your doctor may suggest that you implement certain lifestyle changes before stopping the statin, or directly in place of the drug. These changes might include adopting an exercise program or modifying your diet. For example, the AHATrusted Source suggests following a Mediterranean diet or vegan diet.

Keep in mind, though, that these changes likely won't work as quickly or as effectively as statin in lowering your cholesterol. A healthy diet and exercise program can have many benefits for your overall health, but it may not be enough to replace the cholesterol-lowering effects of a statin.

You and your doctor should closely monitor your cholesterol levels to make sure the diet and exercise changes are having the necessary effects on your cholesterol.

Reducing statin use
Instead of completely stopping your statin use, your doctor might suggest reducing your statin dosage. Less medication could mean fewer side effects, and the drug might still work well enough to manage your cholesterol levels.

Or your doctor could suggest reducing your statin dosage while adding another medication or supplement. This could resolve your issues with taking the drug, especially if they relate to side effects.

Adding other cholesterol drugs

Drugs your doctor could add to your medication regimen while reducing your statin use include ezetimibe, bile acid sequestrants, or niacin. These medications can help manage your cholesterol levels while you take the lower dosage of statins.

Adding L-carnitine supplements

L-carnitine supplements are another option, especially for people with diabetes. L-carnitine is an amino acid derivative made by your body. Preliminary studies have shown that taking L-carnitine twice daily could improve the effect of statins on LDL and also prevent a rise in blood sugar. Learn more about L-carnitine and its effects on the body.

Why you may want to come off statins

Not everyone needs to stop taking statins. Many people take statins for decades without having any side effects or issues. For those individuals, the medications can be a very effective form of treatment and prevention for cholesterol problems.

Others may not have the same experience with statins. People who decide to quit taking statins may have several different reasons for doing so. The following are some of the most common reasons for quitting statins.

Side effects

Statins can cause several side effects. Many of these side effects can be mild, such as muscle pain and cramps. Other side effects can be very severe, such as liver damage, muscle deterioration, and kidney failure.

Mild side effects may be managed, but moderate to severe side effects may become problematic or possibly dangerous. If you and your doctor decide that the danger or damage caused by the statin's side effects outweighs the benefits of the medication, you may need to stop taking it.

Cost

Many types of statins are available today, and most are covered by health insurance plans. However, if you cannot afford to continue taking the statins your doctor prescribed, talk to your doctor. They can help you devise an alternative treatment plan.

Reduced need

Lowering your cholesterol levels through diet, exercise, or weight loss could eliminate your need to take statins or other cholesterol medications. If you can do that, that's great! Reducing your cholesterol levels in this way can help reduce your overall risk of a heart attack, stroke, or blocked arteries while allowing you to take one less medication.

But don't stop taking your statin because you think your cholesterol levels are automatically better because of your lifestyle changes. The only way to know if your cholesterol levels are in a healthy range is with a blood test. Your doctor can give you that test and let you know if you're safe to stop taking your statin.

Talk with your doctor
If you want to stop taking your statin for any reason, talk with your doctor. If your doctor thinks it's safe for you to consider changing your statin usage, they can help guide you. Reducing your dosage, adding supplements, or stopping the drug altogether might all be options.

Overall, the most important thing is to keep your cholesterol levels under control. Stopping statins on your own won't accomplish that goal and could cause serious health risks. Work with your doctor to devise a treatment plan that can meet your cholesterol needs while keeping you safe and healthy.

Chapter 3

Diabetes

How Diabetes Affects Women:

Diabetes can look and feel different for women. Identifying and treating the unique symptoms and risks of women with diabetes may lead to a better quality of life.

Diabetes is a group of metabolic diseases in which a person has high levels of blood glucose — also known as blood sugar — due to problems making or using the hormone insulin. Your body needs insulin to make and use energy from the carbohydrates you consume.

There are three common types:

Type 1 diabetes: Your body can't make insulin due to autoimmune dysfunction.
Type 2 diabetes: This is the most common and occurs when your body is unable to properly use insulin.
Gestational diabetes: This is caused by pregnancy.
Diabetes can affect people with any lifestyle and of any age, race, ethnic group, sex, or gender. The condition can often have more serious effects on women when compared to men.

A 2019 literature reviewTrusted Source looked at the link between diabetes and poor health outcomes in well over 5.1 million people across 49 studies. Researchers found that when compared to men with diabetes, women with diabetes experienced:

13% greater risk of death from all causes
30% greater risk of death from cardiovascular disease
58% greater risk of death from coronary heart disease
Read on to learn more about diabetes in women.

Language matters
We use "women" and "men" in this article to reflect the terms that have been historically used to gender people. However, your gender identity may not align with how your body may respond to diabetes.

A doctor can better help you understand your risk for diabetes and how to manage certain symptoms or complications if you develop the condition.

Was this helpful?

Symptoms of diabetes in women

Women and men with diabetes may experience many of the same symptoms.

However, some symptoms are unique to women. Understanding these symptoms may help you identify diabetes and get treatment for it early.

Candida infections
Hyperglycemia, or high blood sugar levels, can trigger the growth of fungus.

An overgrowth of yeast caused by the Candida fungus can result in vaginal or oral yeast infections. These common infections are also known as thrush.

When an infection develops in the vaginal area, symptoms can include:

vaginal itching
vaginal discharge
painful sex
soreness
Oral yeast infections often cause a white coating on the tongue and inside the mouth.

Urinary tract infections (UTIs)
Urinary tract infections (UTIs) develop when bacteria enter the urinary tract.

The risk is higher in women who have diabetes. UTIs are common in this group mainly because hyperglycemia compromises the immune system.

UTIs can cause:

painful urination
a burning sensation during urination
bloody or cloudy urine
There's a risk of kidney infection if these symptoms aren't treated.

Vaginal dryness
Diabetic neuropathy occurs when high blood sugar levels damage your nerve fibers. This damage can trigger tingling and loss of feeling in different parts of the body, including the:

hands
feet
legs
Diabetic neuropathy may also affect sensation in the vaginal area, leading to symptoms like vaginal dryness.

Polycystic ovary syndrome (PCOS)
Experts don't know the exact cause of polycystic ovary syndrome (PCOS).

It can occur when a woman produces a high amount of androgens (male hormones) and has certain risk factors, such as a family history of PCOS. In one study, researchers found that the main androgens involved in PCOS are testosterone and androstenedione.

Symptoms of PCOS include:

irregular periods
weight gain
acne
depression
infertility
PCOS is also associated with a type of insulin resistance that elevates blood sugar levels and increases your risk of developing diabetes. Insulin resistance may be either a symptom or a cause of PCOS.

Symptoms of diabetes
The following symptoms can potentially affect anyone with diabetes:

increased thirst and hunger
frequent urination
weight loss or weight gain with no obvious cause
fatigue
nausea
blurry vision
wounds that heal slowly
skin infections
acanthosis nigricans, or patches of darker skin at the armpits, groin, and back of the neck
irritability
breath that has a sweet, fruity, or acetone-like odor
reduced feeling in the hands or feet
However, keep in mind that many people with type 2 diabetes have no noticeable symptoms at all.

Pregnancy for people with type 1 or type 2 diabetes:

Type 1 diabetes typically starts during childhood. Type 2 diabetes typically starts in adulthood. If you have one of these conditions before you're pregnant, it's known as pregestational diabetes.

You may wonder if pregnancy is safe if you have pregestational diabetes.

You can certainly have a healthy pregnancy after getting a diagnosis of type 1 diabetes or type 2 diabetes. However, it's important to manage your condition before and during pregnancy to avoid complications.

Your blood sugar levels and general health need to be tracked before and during pregnancy. Talk with your doctor about the best ways to manage your and your baby's health.

If you're planning to get pregnant, it's best to get your blood sugar levels as close to your target range as possible beforehand. Your target blood sugar ranges when pregnant may be different from the ranges when you're not pregnant.

When you're pregnant, blood sugar and ketones travel through the placenta to the baby. Babies require energy from sugar just like you do, but they're at risk for congenital abnormalities if their blood sugar levels are too high.

Transferring high blood sugar to unborn babies puts them at risk for:

premature birth
cognitive impairments
developmental delays
Gestational diabetes
Gestational diabetes occurs when people begin to have high blood sugar during pregnancy. It's different from type 1 and type 2 diabetes.

Gestational diabetes affects almost 10% of pregnancies in the United States, according to the American Diabetes Association (ADA).

Pregnancy hormones interfere with the way insulin works, causing the body to make more insulin. For some people, this still isn't enough insulin, and they develop gestational diabetes.

Gestational diabetes often develops later in pregnancy. Your doctor may test you for it between weeks 24 and 28Trusted Source. For most people, gestational diabetes goes away after pregnancy.

If you've had gestational diabetes, your risk for type 2 diabetes increases. Your doctor may recommend diabetes and prediabetes testing every few years.

Risk factors for diabetes in women
Most people with type 1 diabetes develop the condition in childhood. Risk factors include having a parent or sibling with the condition. Coming from a cold climate may also raise your risk.

In the United States, people who are white are more likely to develop type 1 diabetes than African American, Hispanic, or Latino people, according to the Centers for Disease Control and Prevention (CDC)Trusted Source.

According to the Department of Health and Human Services's Office on Women's HealthTrusted Source, you're at risk for type 2 diabetes if you:

are at least 45 years old
have overweight or obesity
have a parent or sibling with diabetes
are African American, Hispanic, Asian American, American Indian, Alaska Native, Native Hawaiian, or Pacific Islander
have had a baby with a birth weight of at least 9 pounds (4.08 kilograms)
have had gestational diabetes
have high blood pressure
have high cholesterol
are physically active fewer than three times a week
have PCOS
have a history of heart disease or stroke
ResearchersTrusted Source is still exploring the exact reasons why some ethnic and racial groups have a higher risk of type 2 diabetes.

Possible factors may include but aren't limited to:

biological risk factors, such as weight status and the location of fat deposits on the body
lack of access to healthcare
inequities in healthcare
socioeconomic status or other social determinants of health
cultural attitudes and behaviors toward diabetes prevention
Diabetes by the numbers
According to the National Diabetes Statistics ReportTrusted Source, an estimated 37.3 million people (11.3% of the U.S. population) had diabetes in 2019. This includes 19.1 million men and 18.0 million women 18 years or older with the condition.

The World Health Organization (WHO)Trusted Source states that there were 422 million adults globally living with diabetes in 2014, up from 108 million reported in 1980.

The International Diabetes Federation provides global prevalence estimates, among other statistics, in its Diabetes Atlas. In 2021, it predicted that 642.8 million people 20 to 79 years old may have diabetes by 2030. By 2045, 783.7 million people in this age group may have diabetes.

Diabetes treatment:

There's no cure for diabetes. Once you've received the diagnosis, you can only manage your symptoms.

Women may experience unique obstacles to managing their blood sugar and diabetes.

For instance, some birth control pills can increase your blood sugar. To maintain a moderate blood sugar level, ask your doctor about switching to a lplow-dose birth control pill.

Other ways to help manage your diabetes are described below.

Medications
There's a variety of medications you can take to manage symptoms and complications.

Many new classes of diabetes medications are available, but the most common medications for those who have recently received a diagnosis include:

Insulin therapy: Insulin therapy is for all people with type 1 diabetes.
Metformin: Metformin (Fortamet, Glumetza) lowers your blood sugar levels.
Lifestyle changes
Lifestyle changes can also help you manage diabetes. They include:

exercising and maintaining a moderate weight
avoiding smoking cigarettes, if you smoke
following a balanced eating plan that meets your personal needs and is focused on fruits, vegetables, and whole grains
monitoring your blood sugar levels
The ADA's latest consensus report reviewed hundreds of scientific articles on how nutrition and diet can be used to manage diabetes. Researchers found that everyone's body responds differently to foods, including carbohydrates, and there's no single "diabetes diet" that works for all people.

The ADA recommends an individualized approach to eating. This should include working with a registered dietitian to find out what eating plan, macronutrient combination, and food choices make the most sense for your goals.

Alternative remedies
More conclusive research is needed on the benefits of alternative remedies for people with diabetes.

Alternative remedies that may have a slight benefit for people with diabetes include:

supplements like chromium and magnesium
herbs and seeds like buckwheat, sage, and fenugreek seeds
Consult a doctor before trying any new diabetes remedies, even if they're natural. They may interact with your current treatments or medications.

Complications of diabetes
Diabetes can cause a variety of complications, which include:

Eating disorders: According to the ADA, some research suggests that eating disorders are more common in women with diabetes than in women without diabetes.

Coronary heart disease: Many women, even young women, with type 2 diabetes already have heart disease at the time of their diabetes diagnosis.

Skin conditions: Skin-related complications include bacterial and fungal infections.

Nerve damage: Nerve damage can lead to pain, impaired circulation, or loss of feeling in the affected limbs.

Eye damage: Eye damage may lead to vision loss or blindness.

Foot damage: If foot damage isn't treated promptly, it can result in amputation.

Depression: Women with diabetes have a higher risk of depression than men with diabetes and people without diabetes, according to the ADA.

Why diabetes is different for women

There are a few reasons why diabetes affects women differently than it does others:

Women often receive less aggressive treatment for cardiovascular risk factors and diabetes-related conditions.

Women often have different kinds of heart disease than men. Diabetes is also more likely to raise a woman's risk of heart disease than a man's, according to the Centers for Disease Control and Prevention (CDC)Trusted Source.

Some diabetes complications are more difficult to diagnose in women.

Hormones and inflammation act differently in women.

Chapter 4

Healthy aging

When many people think of growing older and aging, they often associate many negative thoughts with the aging process. However, it's important to recognize that a lot of these preconceived notions are passed down to us through social conditioning and broader culture from TV, books, and movies. However, Vincent Giampapa, M.D. and Nobel Prize winner for his innovative research on cellular restoration technology says that having a positive mindset and belief system toward aging is one of the keys to a healthy aging formula.

Additionally, the National Institute of Health says some of the most important components of healthy aging and wellness are targeting blood pressure, lowering cholesterol, exercising regularly, and avoiding alcohol and smoking.

In this article, we'll reveal the top science-backed 10 secrets of healthy aging so you can have a good quality of life no matter your age.

1. Aerobic Exercise
There are countless benefits to having aerobic exercise as a regular part of your healthy aging formula, including:

Slowing down the body's aging process
Reducing risks of stress, depression, and hardened arteries.
Improving muscle and bone health
Keeping muscles flexible
Producing higher levels of endorphins and serotonin to improve overall mood and brain function
Improving sleep function
Maintain a steady weight
Not only is aerobic exercise proven to delay biological aging, but it can also help you live longer, and you don't need to be a high-performing marathon runner to reap the benefits. Exercise can come in the form of gardening, regularly walking a dog, going for short jogs, taking an aerobic exercise class a few times a week, and many more.

2. Incorporate the right ingredients into your diet
What you choose to put into your body has a huge, lasting impact on healthy aging and wellness. 'Whole foods' has become a bit of a buzzword as of late, but this is more of a way of eating as opposed to a strict diet. When you fill your body every day with whole grains, nuts, fruits, and vegetables, you can live longer and reduce your body's risk of getting diseases and ailments such as heart disease, cancer, Parkinson's, and more.

Probiotics

Probiotics can be found in fermented foods and drinks such as kimchi, yogurt, kombucha, sauerkraut, and more. Probiotics are live cultures that can influence the chemistry of the bacteria in your gut. While the benefits of probiotics at times have been exaggerated, many dieticians and doctors recommend having them implemented as a regular part of your diet to contribute to healthy aging in women.

However, if you're considering introducing more probiotics into your diet, speak with your doctor, particularly if you're currently taking any antibiotics, in which case probiotics may produce an adverse effect.

Fish
Eating several servings of fish each week is important for healthy aging and wellness. The high amounts of omega-3s found in different types of fish can help lower the risk of heart disease and your chances of having a heart attack. The American Heart Association encourages fish and omega-3 fatty acids as a regular staple in a person's diet for those at higher risk of cardiovascular disease and also to help in keeping blood pressure low.

As far as aging goes, the EPA and DHA found in fatty fish can combat muscular degeneration, which can lead to blindness in older groups.

Potassium
Eating a lot of potassium-rich foods like fruits, bananas, tomatoes, potatoes, and more is another great way to implement healthy aging through diet. Potassium helps you develop lean muscle tissue, which begins to decrease naturally in your body at around age 65. Too much loss of muscle mass can lead to serious health issues, so make sure you're getting the proper daily dose of 4.7 grams.

Vitamin B (B12)
B12 is commonly found in seafood and poultry products and is known to help keep your energy levels up. This vitamin is not naturally produced by your body, therefore you must find sources of it elsewhere. B12 is also good for:

Preventing anemia
Promoting red blood cell formation
Supporting bone health and preventing osteoporosis
Decreasing your risk of macular degeneration, which affects your vision
Helping combat depression and boosting overall mood
Helping with memory retention
Supporting healthy hair, skin, and nails
A supplement may be a good source of getting the B12 your body needs. For those 65 and older, speak with your doctor as older groups are advised to take B12 as part of a B-complex vitamin because the latter might be too harsh on the stomach.

Vitamin D

Vitamin D is one of the best defenses against age-related diseases like cardiovascular disease, high blood pressure, some cancers, and autoimmune disorders. You can easily get vitamin D from foods like eggs, fish, and milk, but your body also produces vitamin D on its own when exposed to sunlight.

Many people don't get as much vitamin D as they should though, so speak with your doctor about potentially taking a supplement or schedule regular 20-minute intervals per day in the sunlight.

The main takeaway here is that the foods and ingredients you ingest have a real effect on your chromosomes and can combat your risk of age-related diseases. A study conducted by the University of Michigan found that "eating a diet that is rich in fruits, vegetables, and whole grains and low in added sugar, sodium, and processed meats could help promote healthy cellular aging in women."

3. Schedule social time
As human beings, we naturally crave connection and acceptance. Chronic loneliness has been linked to a higher risk of depression, anxiety, and even dementia.

Conversely, according to the National Institute of Aging, people who regularly take part in social activities can boost their mood and they also tend to live longer.

Even if you don't live close to family, you can always engage in volunteer work, casual learning courses, and even connect with loved ones on social networks to help you stay more connected and social in your life.

4. Relaxing exercises like Yoga or Tai Chi
Both Yoga and Tai Chi boast the following benefits:

Improves physical functioning
Lowers blood pressure
Relief from stress and anxiety
Slows down bone loss post-menopause
Aids with experiencing better sleep
Increases flexibility
Improves balance
Lessens pain from arthritis
Both Yoga and Tai Chi are easy to learn and very simple to do many health clubs and community centers offer low-cost or free classes for these types of meditative exercises. Both incorporate slow movement, strength training, and deep breathing practices which aid in overall cognitive function and well-being.

5. Cut back on red meat

High consumption of red meat is linked with multiple health problems. While small amounts per week can be nutritious, eating too much of it can lead to higher cholesterol levels, colorectal cancer, and type 2 diabetes.

Try replacing a few of your red meat dishes in the week with poultry, fish, or even tofu for a healthier balance of red meat in your diet.

6. Reduce your sugar intake
Sugar has been proven to age us both externally in our appearances and internally. With many foods these days containing hidden traces of sugar, it's important to indulge in desserts and sweets now and then, and also be on the lookout for sneaky sources of sugar in foods like granola, yogurt, milk, and juices.

Sugar is also known to damage the liver, make blood pressure levels go up, and change metabolism levels, so make sure that when you add sugar into your diet, you're incorporating it wisely.

7. Use your brain
The belief that our mental abilities inevitably decline as we get older is largely false. While brain chemistry does change as we age, you should keep your brain active the form of taking a fun class, learning a new language, doing a daily crossword puzzle, writing, or engaging in stimulating conversation. These activities will help keep your brain more "young" and alert. As they say, if you don't use it, you lose it!

8. Drink Green Tea
Green tea has strong antioxidants in it that help reduce inflammation in the body and promote overall better aging. Green tea is particularly known for having a high amount of the antioxidant EGCG, which can help increase cell turnover (and helps reduce wrinkles!)

9. Go for your regular checkups
Going in for your normal health examinations is critical to healthy aging so you can be aware of any signs of serious health problems before they become worse. Make sure to go in for regular appointments such as:

Annual physical
This is probably the most common form of physical examination where your vitals are checked (blood pressure, weight, etc.) as well as your blood to see if you're lacking anything or showing signs of potential diseases or other health problems.

As a refresher, we have an article on the 9 most common female health problems you may want to look at for healthy aging and wellness.

Gynecologist

For females, going in for your regular gynecological appointment is vital to female health and wellness. If you're curious about how the gynecologist can help you, we have an article on the top questions for gynecologists answered here.

Dentist
Your risk of gum disease increases as you get older and going in for regular dental appointments in addition to brushing and flossing are the best ways to prevent gum disease. Gum disease and tooth loss are associated with an increased risk of cardiovascular disease. So, make sure you're going in for regular dental checkups and teeth cleanings.

10. Getting regular Mammograms
Mammograms are an x-ray of the breast. This is a regular examination meant to detect breast cancer. Most women are advised to get their first mammogram at around age 40 or 45, and this might be younger for those at a higher risk of developing breast cancer. Make sure you talk with your doctor about when you should start getting regular mammograms.

We have another article all about mammograms where we cover what to expect and clear up commonly asked questions about the procedure.

While aging is an inevitable part of continuing life, at the end of the day, it is all about whether you decide to have a positive or a negative attitude. We hope our article on the 10 secrets to healthy aging has been enlightening for you, so you can begin on the path toward living a full, happy life as you age.

A good way to work positivity into your healthy aging formula is to make sure you reflect on the healthy aspects of aging, such as increased life experience, wisdom, thinking about what you're appreciative of, and everything you've been able to accomplish with the life you've lived so far.

Chapter 5

Heart health

Heart disease is the leading cause of death for women in the United States. Find out what other women like you know about heart health and get tips on how to keep your heart healthy!

Among women, 90% have one or more risk factors for heart disease at some point in their lives, according to American Heart Association statistics. Yet 80% of cardiovascular diseases are preventable.

Get annual checkups

It's important to get annual checkups to assess heart-health risks and take action, Mieres said. Prepare for the appointment, much as you would when gathering documents to meet with a financial adviser.

"You go to your accountant at tax time, and you don't show up empty-handed," she said. Be prepared to discuss any family history of heart disease or other concerns. "You should not be passive. You should have a conversation."

Become knowledgeable of your key health numbers, such as blood pressure, cholesterol, and blood sugar levels. For example, blood pressure of less than 120/80 is considered normal.

Know the symptoms of a heart attack

Women's heart attack symptoms may cover a wider spectrum compared with symptoms in men. Women may experience the "classic" heart attack symptoms of chest pressure, chest discomfort, or shortness of breath, just as men do.

"But women also may have symptoms such as back pain, usually on the left side; shoulder pain; a fullness in the stomach; or nausea as signs of an impending heart attack," cautioned Mieres.

Tell your doctor if you had a pregnancy complication

Recent research has focused on heart disease linked to pregnancy-related complications. Diabetes and hypertension during pregnancy, as well as early delivery, have been linked to increased cardiovascular disease risk years later.

"Pregnancy is a stress test" for the body, a possible marker for heart disease later in life, said Mieres.

Get enough sleep

Lack of sleep – getting less than six or seven hours a night – is connected to heart disease, research has shown. Poor sleep has been linked to high blood pressure, can make it difficult to lose weight, and may make you less likely to want to exercise.

Tame stress

Chronic stress is another area of concern for women. It can lead to behaviors and factors that impact heart disease, such as high blood pressure, high cholesterol, inactivity, and overeating.

To cope with stress, eat healthy foods, exercise, and get plenty of sleep. Consider talking to others about your stress, including a friend, parent, doctor, or counselor.

Find a health partner

In all heart-healthy efforts, it helps to have a partner in the endeavor, Mieres said.

Work with a healthcare provider to find a customized treatment plan that fits your daily life and medical needs. A friend, family member, or co-worker also can be a good partner for getting physically active and sticking with a healthy eating plan.

"It's OK if you fall off the wagon. You have that person to help you get back on track," said Mieres. "There is strength in numbers."

If you have questions or comments about this story, please email editor@heart.org.

Other uses, including educational products or services sold for profit, must comply with the American Heart Association's Copyright Permission Guidelines. See full terms of use. These stories may not be used to promote or endorse a commercial product or service.

Thanks to ongoing advances in medicine and a relatively high standard of living, most women in the United States today can look forward to living well into their late 70s or early 80s. But while you may enjoy a greater life expectancy than your mother, grandmother, or great-grandmother did, a longer life doesn't necessarily mean a healthier one.

It's precisely because you can expect to live longer that you should do everything in your power to ensure you're as healthy as possible. But what, exactly, does that mean?

Here at Women's Healthcare of Princeton, we believe that good health is more than just a concept — it's a lifelong commitment to mindful action. Making healthy lifestyle changes at any time, whether you're in your 20s, 40s, or 60s, can help you avoid chronic illness and slow down the aging process, inside and out.

In celebration of National Women's Health Week, we offer six of our best tips for taking steps toward personal optimal health, no matter where you are in life.

Be physically active more often
It's hard to overstate the importance of regular physical activity. In general, women who exercise tend to have healthier blood pressure and cholesterol levels and also have a lower risk of developing serious chronic illnesses like heart disease, diabetes, and dementia. As you approach menopause, staying physically active can also help curtail or alleviate bothersome symptoms like hot flashes, night sweats, and moodiness.

Finding the time for 30-60 minutes of moderate-intensity exercise most days of the week can help you sleep better, give you more energy, help control unhealthy food cravings, and keep you at a healthy body weight.

Easier said than done, right? Fortunately, there are easy and practical ways to boost your activity level. Simply getting a fitness tracker can give you the motivation to increase your daily step count. To make it even more interesting, try challenging your friends and coworkers to weekly step competitions.

Take the stairs as often as possible to work more activity into your day, or work in more steps by routinely parking your car a little further away from your destination. Walking is a great way to get centered, decompress, or enjoy the weather, too. Go for an early morning walk before you head to work, or just after you get home before you wind down for the evening.

If you're already active, chances are you can find ways to improve your fitness routine. A well-rounded exercise program places as much emphasis on strength and endurance as it does on flexibility, balance, and mobility.

Make sleep a top priority
For many women, the demands of modern life make it increasingly harder to get a good night's sleep. But here's the thing: Your to-do list isn't nearly as important as the health benefits that quality sleep can provide.

Getting the amount of sleep you need to feel rested and balanced can help you stay productive, preserve a higher level of reasoning, and keep your emotions steady. It also helps protect your long-term health.

Sleep is an important factor at all stages of life. It's restorative for mind and body alike. Women who routinely don't get enough sleep are more likely to have weight control issues and memory problems — plus an increased risk of developing heart disease.

Start by cultivating better sleep habits. Don't consume caffeine after 2 pm. Avoid screen time within 30 minutes of going to bed — put your phone on silent or in sleep mode and turn off all alerts. Instead of watching TV or using a computer or tablet, read a book or listen to relaxing music.

You may find it helpful to use meditative practices and deep breathing to clear your mind or try bedtime journaling to release any thoughts that are weighing you down.

Schedule an annual well-woman exam
If you only see your doctor when you're not feeling well, you're missing out on a major chance to safeguard your long-term health. You can't take care of an underlying health problem if you don't know about it.

Preventive care is a cornerstone of good health, and that means you're never too busy to make time for your annual well-woman exam. It's an excellent opportunity to check for serious health concerns that typically go unnoticed, including high blood pressure and unhealthy cholesterol levels. It's also a good time to evaluate your need for a mammogram, Pap test, HPV screening, and osteoporosis screening.

Quit smoking for good
Smoking is a devastating habit that harms every bodily system. Besides increasing your risk for various types of cancer, it also makes you more likely to develop osteoporosis, rheumatoid arthritis, cataracts, and gum disease. Women who smoke are also more likely to go through menopause at an earlier age than those who don't.

Come in for a visit to talk with us about ways you can quit smoking for good. Know that you're not alone — tobacco addiction affects 14% of American women — but there are support groups, medications, and substitutes that can help. The good news is that quitting smoking, even if you've already reached middle age, can cut your risk of early death in half.

Improve your diet
Pay attention to what you're eating! Eating healthy doesn't mean bland food. On the contrary, it can mean fresh and fun flavors, colorful appetizing plates, and a whole new world of ingredients you've never tried before. Try to eat whole, fresh foods as often as possible. Even when time doesn't permit a home-cooked meal, take a look at the ingredients in the packaged foods you buy at the store.

Pay particular attention to sugar and carbohydrate content, especially in foods that are labeled "low-fat." Consider whole-grain or vegetarian alternatives that are less processed and more nutritious — faro, quinoa, or cauliflower rice are healthier alternatives to white rice and traditional pasta, for example. Add herbs and spices to expand flavors and make healthy meals more interesting.

Put more fiber in your diet, which is found in plant-based foods like vegetables, legumes, fruits, whole grains, nuts, and seeds. Women who eat a fiber-rich diet are more likely to maintain a lower body weight, avoid chronic illness, and live longer.

Escape the monotony of daily routine
When you have a lot going on in your life, having a solid routine can help you get through the day with greater ease. But when your routine starts to feel like a rut, you can lose touch with yourself.

To stimulate your mind and bring a little creative energy back into your life, try shaking things up. Turn off your phone, and give yourself 20 minutes each day to engage in something you love. Whether you choose to meditate, head outside for a walk, paint a picture, or spend a few minutes learning a new language, your 20-minute moment will reinvigorate your mind for the rest of the day.

As women's health experts, there's nothing more exciting for us than being able to help you find your best personal wellness. Let us know how we can help you. Call our office in Princeton, New Jersey, or schedule an appointment online at any time.

Pay attention to what you're eating! Eating healthy doesn't mean boring or bland food. On the contrary, it can mean fresh and fun flavors, colorful appetizing plates, and a whole new world of ingredients you've never tried before. Try to eat whole, fresh foods as often as possible. Even when time doesn't permit a home-cooked meal, take a look at the ingredients in the packaged foods you buy at the store.

Pay particular attention to sugar and carbohydrate content, especially in foods that are labeled "low-fat." Consider whole-grain or vegetarian alternatives that are less processed and more nutritious — faro, quinoa, or cauliflower rice are healthier alternatives to white rice and traditional pasta, for example. Add herbs and spices to expand flavors and make healthy meals more interesting.

Put more fiber in your diet, which is found in plant-based foods like vegetables, legumes, fruits, whole grains, nuts, and seeds. Women who eat a fiber-rich diet are more likely to maintain a lower body weight, avoid chronic illness, and live longer.

Escape the monotony of daily routine
When you have a lot going on in your life, having a solid routine can help you get through the day with greater ease. But when your routine starts to feel like a rut, you can lose touch with yourself.

To stimulate your mind and bring a little creative energy back into your life, try shaking things up. Turn off your phone, and give yourself 20 minutes each day to engage in something you love. Whether you choose to meditate, head outside for a walk, paint a picture, or spend a few minutes learning a new language, your 20-minute moment will reinvigorate your mind for the rest of the day.

As women's health experts, there's nothing more exciting for us than being able to help you find your best personal wellness. Let us know how we can help you. Call our office in Princeton, New Jersey, or schedule an appointment online any time.